PRESTON COLLEGE
WILLIAM TUSON LIBRARY
with draw

10853577

Ingredients of a Balanced Diet

Grains

Rachel Eugster

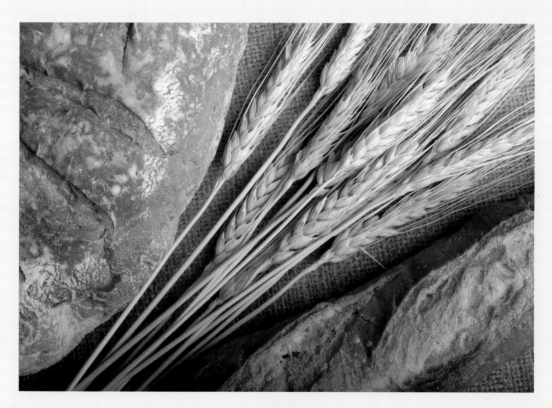

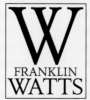

FRANKLIN
WATTS

First published in 2007 by
Franklin Watts
338 Euston Road,
London NW1 3BH

Franklin Watts Australia
Hachette Children's Books
Level 17/207 Kent Street
Sydney NSW 2000

© 2007 Bender Richardson White
All rights reserved

INGREDIENTS OF A BALANCED DIET:
GRAINS was produced for Franklin Watts by
Bender Richardson White, PO Box 266,
Uxbridge, UK.
Editor and Picture Researcher: Lionel Bender
Designer and Page Make-up: Ben White
Cover Make-up: Mike Pilley, Radius
Production: Kim Richardson
Graphics and Maps: Stefan Chabluk

A CIP catalogue record for this book is
available from the British Library.

ISBN: 978 0 7496 6801 3
Dewey classification: 641.3

Printed in China

Note to parents and teachers: Every effort has
been made by the Publishers to ensure that the
websites in this book are suitable for children,
that they are of the highest educational value,
and that they contain no inappropriate or
offensive material. However, because of the
nature of the Internet, it is impossible to
guarantee that the contents of these sites will
not be altered. We strongly advise that Internet
access is supervised by a responsible adult.

Franklin Watts is a division of Hachette
Children's Books

Picture credits

Bubbles Photo Library: pages 26 and 27 (John
Powell). foodanddrinkphotos.com: pages 7, 9, 16,
17, 19, 21. iStockphotos: pages 1, 3, 30, 31, 32
and all Food bite panels (Peter Clark); pages 1 and
12 (Donald Gruener); page 3 and all Recipe boxes
(Amanda Rohde); pages 4 (Andrea Gingerich); 5
(Monika Adamczyk); 10 (Edyta Pawlowska); 11
(Natalia Clarke); 14 (Carmen Martinez); 15 (P.
Wei); 18 (Stephen Orsillo); 20 (Chaleerat
Ngamchalee); 23 (KMITU); 24 (aabejon).
Cover image: foodanddrinkphotos.com.
BRW wishes to thank Sarah Bell and colleagues at
foodanddrinkphotos.com for setting up the
commissioned photography.

The author
Rachel Eugster is a food, health and
nutrition writer and editor. Formerly food
editor of *Walking* magazine, she is a
regular contributor to *Continental* and
YES Mag and creates recipes for people of
all ages. She feeds her family as healthy a
diet as they will eat!

The consultant
Ester Davies is a professional food and
nutrition writer, lecturer and consultant.
She has a B.Ed. in Food, Nutrition and
Sociology. She has written books on food
specifically for the National Curriculum.

Note: In recipes, liquid measures and small
quantities are given by volume in millilitres
(ml) as this is how measuring jugs and
spoons are usually marked.

Contents

Food for life 4

Food groups and diet 6

Grains, fibre and vitamins 8

Getting to know grains 10

An amazing variety 12

How grains are eaten 14

Meals with grains 16

Vegetarian meals 18

Cooking and serving 20

Digestion 22

Energy balance 24

Shopping and storing 26

Projects 28

Glossary 30

Websites 31

Index 32

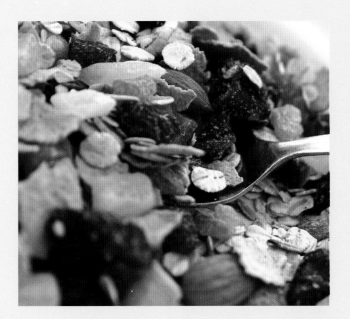

Food for life

Grains are the edible seeds of grasses. They are also known as cereals. Grains include wheat, oats, barley and rice. They are eaten on their own and are used to make a variety of foods ranging from breakfast cereals to pastas, noodles, breads, tortillas, crackers, biscuits and cakes.

Nutrients

Foods and drinks contain nutrients, which are materials your body needs but cannot make itself. Nutrients allow your body to work properly, to stay healthy and active, and to grow. Grains are good sources of nutrients such as carbohydrates, B vitamins, minerals and fibre. Try and eat about 75g of grains or grain products each day. This is roughly the amount of grain in three slices of wholemeal bread, a large bowl of breakfast cereal or a bowl of cooked rice, cooked pasta or cooked cereal.

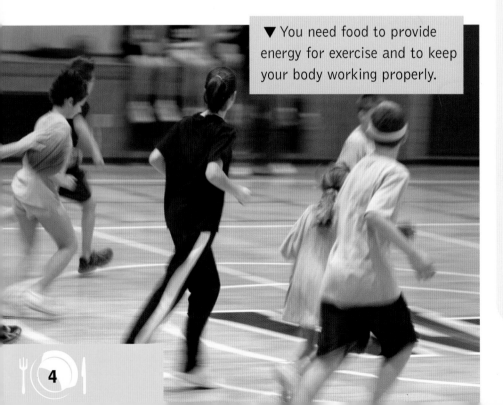

▼ You need food to provide energy for exercise and to keep your body working properly.

Nutrition facts

Major nutrients

Sugars and starches, or carbohydrates: give you energy for walking, talking, playing – even for eating! Fibre is a kind of carbohydrate that helps digestion.

Proteins: needed to make and repair cells and tissues, the building materials of your body.

Vitamins and minerals: help you fight disease, digest food and strengthen your bones and teeth. (See pages 8–9 for more details.)

Fats: store energy for later use, and carry vitamins to where they are needed. Unsaturated fats – those from plant foods – are better for you than saturated fats – which are in meat and dairy products.

Keeping a balance

What you eat and drink, and how much, is your diet. A balanced diet gives you everything you need and is low in unhealthy foods, such as certain fats, sugars and salt. Grains and grain products should form about one-third of your diet. If you eat them together with a wide range of other foods – and do a good deal of exercise – you should stay healthy and fit.

Energy

Foods and drinks contain energy, too. You need energy to make your muscles work. The energy in foods is measured in kilocalories or kilojoules. Compared to other foods, grains contain medium levels of energy. You will need more kilocalories when you are active and playing sport than when you are studying, reading or sleeping. Energy you do not use up is stored in your body as fat. You can find out more about food and energy on pages 24 and 25.

▼ Grains of rice. In the middle are rice grains with chaff. To the left are whole grains and to the right are 'refined' grains.

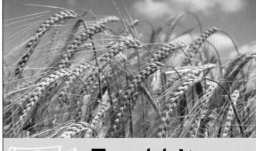

Food bites

Grains are seeds

Grains are well wrapped. We do not eat the outermost layer, called chaff. Beneath this is a layer known as the bran. Inside the bran are the germ and endosperm.

Whole grains include the bran, germ and endosperm. Whole grains are rich in carbohydrates (including fibre), proteins, minerals and vitamins. 'Wholemeal' is a type of flour made from whole grains (see page 10). 'Refined' grains have had the bran and germ removed.

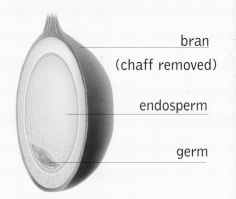

bran
(chaff removed)

endosperm

germ

Water

Water is an important nutrient. You cannot survive more than a few days without it. From your food, you get about half of the 2 litres of water your body needs each day. The rest you must drink. Grains are about 10% water.

Almost everything that goes on inside your body depends upon water. It:

- helps you digest your food
- helps move nutrients to where they are needed
- keeps you cool (that is why you sweat when you exercise)
- lubricates your skeleton joints and protects your brain and eyes
- contains no calories.

Food groups and diet

Foods are often sorted into groups based on the nutrients they provide. Grains are part of a group that are good sources of carbohydrates, vitamins and minerals. To help you know what and how much to eat from each group, food scientists have created diagrams like the food pyramid and food plate shown below. On the food pyramid, for example, the larger the level on the diagram, the more of those foods you should eat. The diagrams show you should eat some unsaturated fats but avoid saturated fats.

Food pyramid and food plate

A food pyramid Eat more from the bottom level – which includes grains – and less from the upper levels.

A food plate One quarter is protein-rich foods, three-quarters are a mix of grains, fruits and vegetables.

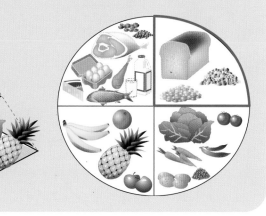

The three-quarter rule

A first step to building a balanced diet is to imagine that your plate is divided into four equal sections. Fill one quarter with protein-rich red meat, poultry, fish, nuts, pulses or dairy products. Fill the other three quarters with other foods. These can be vegetables, salad, brown rice, potatoes, bread or pasta — any food from the larger sections on the food plate or pyramid. This change in filling your plate can make a big difference in your diet.

Go for grains

When choosing grain foods, go for wholegrain whenever possible. This will give you the maximum benefit of the nutrients in grains. Wholegrain breakfast cereals, brown rice, bulgur – also known as cracked wheat – whole wheat pasta and wholemeal bread are all good choices and are widely available in shops.

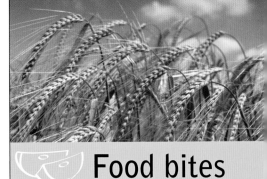

Food bites

Main food groups

1. Bread and other grain products, and potatoes.
2. Fruits and vegetables.
3. Milk and dairy products.
4. Meat, seafood, eggs, seeds, nuts and pulses.
5. Fatty, sugary and salty foods.

▼ Sandwiches made with wholemeal bread are good for including grains in your diet. Fill them with anything you like, including salad, meat, fish, egg or cheese.

Grains, fibre and vitamins

Grains are rich in several minerals. These include calcium needed for healthy bones and teeth; iron essential for healthy red blood cells and brain cells; and magnesium needed for chemical reactions in your body. Grains are also good sources of B vitamins, which help unlock the energy from your food.

Grains also contain proteins for body growth and repair. In general, they contain little of the things that people should avoid in their diet, such as saturated fat, salt and sugar.

Nutrition facts

Vitamin needs

Vitamin A for healthy eyes, blood and bones

B vitamins to prevent heart disease and some cancers

Vitamin C to prevent blood vessel disorders and fight infections

Vitamin D for healthy bones and to prevent cancer

Vitamin E to prevent cell damage

Vitamin K for healthy blood and bones

Nutrient levels

A comparison of the nutrient content of various foods. The lengths of the sections show the percentage of each nutrient in each food. The bars highlight that grains and grain products are rich in carbohydrates and low in fats.

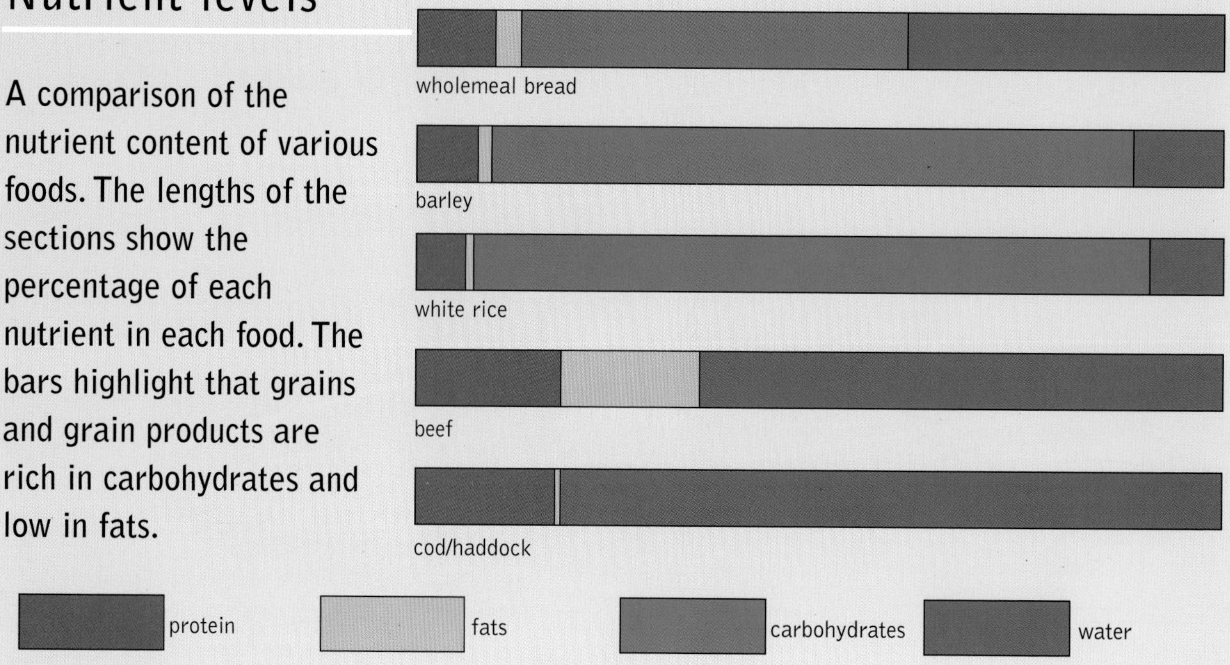

wholemeal bread

barley

white rice

beef

cod/haddock

protein   fats   carbohydrates   water

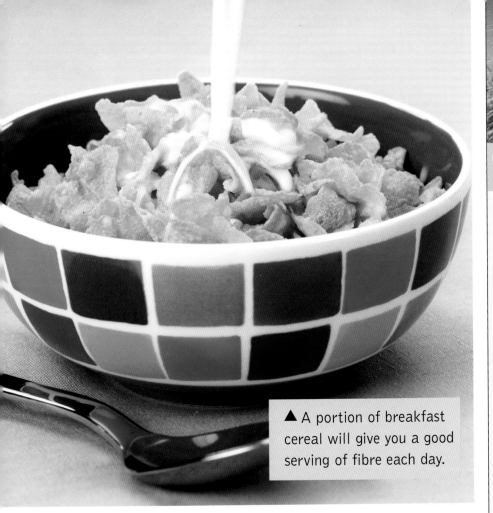

▲ A portion of breakfast cereal will give you a good serving of fibre each day.

Fibre

One very important nutrient is something you cannot even digest. Fibre is found only in plant foods, and whole cereal grains such as brown rice are very good sources of a kind called insoluble fibre. Insoluble means it does not dissolve in water. This type of fibre helps your body get rid of the bits from food that it cannot use, just the way a broom sweeps out rubbish. Getting rid of undigested food keeps your digestive system in good working order.

More help with digestion

The other kind of fibre is called soluble – some of it dissolves in water, making a jelly-like substance that also helps digestion by removing unwanted material. Good grain sources of soluble fibre are oats and barley.

Food bites

Starchy foods

Carbohydrates in grains and other foods are made of sugar molecules. Starch is a mixture of sugars. Many plants store sugars as starch.

Why can you eat more starchy foods like pasta than, say, a beefburger before you feel full up? Because starchy foods are digested in your stomach more quickly than fatty foods, and you can use up the energy in them almost straight away. Also, fatty foods contain roughly twice as many kilocalories as starchy foods. For the same weights, brown rice has half as many kilocalories as a grilled beefburger, about one-third as many as roast chicken, and about one-fifth as many as potato crisps.

Flour

Grains are the main source of flour, which we mix with water and other ingredients to make bread and pasta. Flour is also known as meal. The grains are ground a lot to make fine, soft, powdery flour or a little to make coarse flour. You can buy all-purpose flour, bread flour, cake or pastry flour.

Nutrition facts

Healthier bread

Compared with white bread, wholemeal bread has:
- 7.5% fewer calories
- 7.7% more fat (the good kind from plants)
- 26.9% more protein
- 287.5% more fibre.

Getting to know grains

You probably already eat a lot of grains, in breads, pastas, pizza and baked foods. You may have white rice fairly often, too, perhaps with a curry or as rice pudding. Your biggest grain meal of the day might be breakfast – cereals, porridge or muesli. Scones, crumpets and pancakes contain grains too.

While you may eat grains frequently, they may not be in their best form. For example, cake is mostly flour, which is made from wheat. But most cake flour has

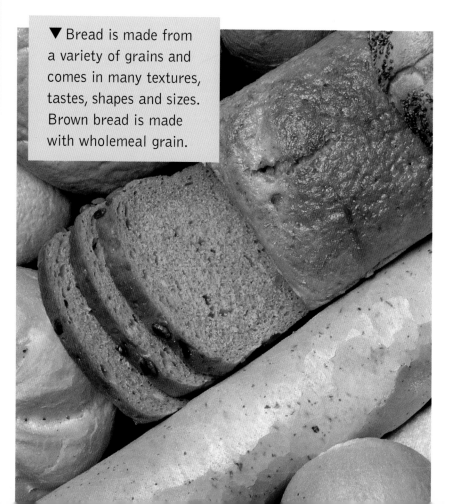

▼ Bread is made from a variety of grains and comes in many textures, tastes, shapes and sizes. Brown bread is made with wholemeal grain.

been refined. That means that the bran and the germ were removed before the wheat was made into flour. This helps the flour keep better, but it also reduces the nutritional value. Also, to make a cake, a lot of saturated fat and sugar is usually added. A piece of cake is a tasty treat, but you cannot build a healthy, balanced diet on it. It contains many 'empty calories' – kilocalories that are not combined with good nutrients.

Upgrading what you eat

Replacing some of the refined grains you eat with whole grains will automatically improve your diet. Choose wholemeal bread instead of white. Try whole brown rice instead of white rice. If you like to bake, add a little wholemeal flour or wheat germ instead of using only white all-purpose flour. This is an excellent second step towards building a balanced diet.

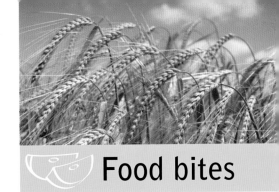

Food bites

Pasta

Pasta is made and eaten worldwide. It is usually made from durum wheat flour and water, but other flours can be used. Vegetable oil or egg may be added. The pasta dough is pushed through machines and made into many different shapes. In Asia, long, flat strips of pasta are called noodles (see page 15).

Dried pasta will keep well for months and comes in many shapes. Fresh pasta must be eaten sooner. Pasta can be flavoured with vegetables, herbs and spices, seafood, fruit – or even chocolate.

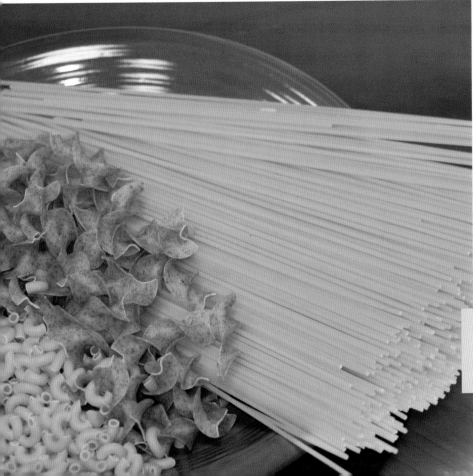

◀ Pasta includes spaghetti and macaroni. It is a popular Italian food, often eaten with meat sauce.

An amazing variety

How many grains can you name? Wheat, rice, oats, rye and barley are probably familiar. Less common but often used grains are triticale, maize, amaranth, millet, quinoa and sorghum. Each type of grain comes in different forms. Roughly 40,000 different types of rice are grown around the world. These can have long, medium or short grains, and include such varieties as basmati, arborio, jasmine and sticky rice.

Half the world's population depends upon rice as a major part of its diet. Rice can be eaten whole, ground into flour or even made into drinks.

Nutrition facts

Genetically modified food

Food scientists can now transfer genes – the hereditary material of living things – from one plant to another. This can increase the nutrients in grains, kill weeds and reduce the need for pesticides.

New varieties of grains produced in this way can provide new types of flour and vegetable oils. But some people are against changing nature and worry that these genetically modified (GM) foods may cause unexpected problems.

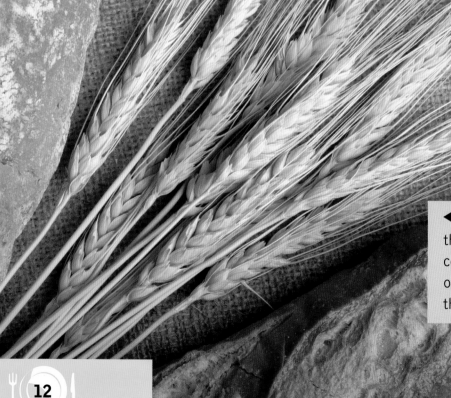

◀ Grains are produced on long, thin spikes or 'ears' at the top of cereal plants. The ears are beaten or rubbed – a process called threshing – to release the grains.

Less familiar grains

Triticale is a cross between wheat and rye. Wild rice is a grass but not a form of rice. Maize comes as corn-on-the-cob and as sweetcorn. Buckwheat and millet are now common grains, but amaranth and chia – once eaten by the Aztecs of Mexico – and quinoa – an ancient grain of the Incas of Peru – are not used widely. Each grain offers a different package of nutrients.

Where in the world?

The origins of grains, and where they are staple diets.

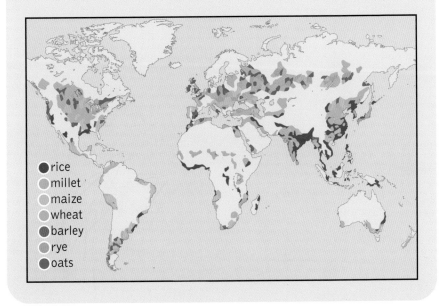

- ● rice
- ● millet
- ● maize
- ● wheat
- ● barley
- ● rye
- ● oats

Staple foods

In much of Asia and Africa, grains are the staple food, which means they form the main part of people's diet. In these continents, rice, millet and sorghum are the main grains. More people in the world eat rice every day than any other food. Bread is one grain food eaten all round the world. Grains are also the world's main source of food for farm animals.

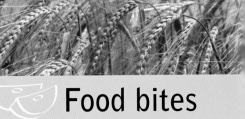

Food bites

Growing grains

Corn is the name some farmers use for the main cereal crop they grow, whether it is wheat, oats or barley. Corn is also a name used for the grains of the maize plant.

More grains are grown around the world and provide more energy to humans than any other kind of food crop. Grains are eaten in a variety of ways:

- Oats can be eaten machine-rolled to soften them or ground into flour.
- Maize meal is used like flour or to make a thick mush known as polenta.
- Hominy is a wholegrain maize dish from the south of the USA.
- Rye is eaten as flakes or used in the form of flour.

Quick quinoa-mince stir-fry

Makes 6 servings.

Ingredients
480ml water
200g quinoa
500g lean mince meat
2 400-g tins of chopped tomatoes, drained
5ml oregano
5ml basil
pepper to taste

Preparation
Bring the water and quinoa to the boil in a saucepan. Lower the heat, cover the pan and simmer for 15 minutes. Or cook the quinoa according to the packet instructions.

Meanwhile, cook the mince in a frying pan, stirring frequently, until done. Add the tomatoes, oregano, basil, pepper and cooked quinoa.

Stir well, cook until heated through, then serve.

▶ Paella is usually made with long-grain rice but noodles can be used. Shellfish, meat and vegetables are baked or steamed over the rice until they are done.

How grains are eaten

People eat grains around the world in more ways you can count. Think of all the different ways you eat rice: with curries, in casseroles, soups, salads and puddings – even in cereals and snacks. In Italy, rice is cooked into a creamy dish called risotto, flavoured with anything from mushrooms to sausages and wine. Paella is very popular in Spain. It is a mixture of rice, shellfish, sausage, chicken and vegetables. In Asia, rice is made into many kinds of noodles and wraps. These dishes are now eaten here.

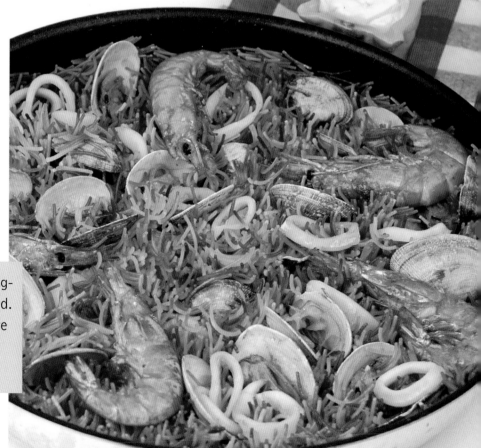

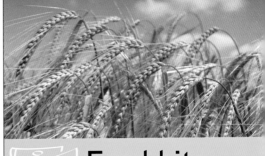

Nutrition facts

Bread

Grains of wheat, oat, maize, rye and barley are all used to make bread. The flour from each grain gives a special flavour, texture and colour to the bread. The flour is mixed with water or milk, oil, salt and often egg to make bread dough. Yeast – a type of fungus – or baking powder may be added to create bubbles of gas that make the dough rise, forming leavened bread. Flat, or unleavened, bread has no raising agent.

Millet, amaranth and barley

Millet can be eaten as a side dish, in stews and in puddings. In Africa, it is cooked in water (like rice), made into porridges and turned into beer. Amaranth is widely used in South America. Rice, millet and amaranth can be sweetened and eaten with dried fruit for breakfast.

Barley is most often found in soups. But it, too, can be eaten like rice as a dish with meat and a thick sauce. In Ireland, it is cooked into an apple pudding.

Quinoa, kamut and wild rice

Quinoa and kamut – a type of wheat – can be eaten hot or used in salads. Try making rice salad or a stir-fry – see the recipe opposite – using quinoa. For a Greek type of salad, toss cold cooked kamut with feta cheese, olives, green peppers and tomatoes.

Wild rice can be used just like white or brown rice, or mixed with them half and half. Wild rice is delicious in stuffed peppers, or in stuffed chicken or turkey instead of breadcrumbs.

Food bites

Noodles

Noodles are made not only from various types of wheat flour but also from rice and mung bean flour. Egg is often added to the flour. Some recently discovered noodles, 4,000 years old, were millet noodles from China.

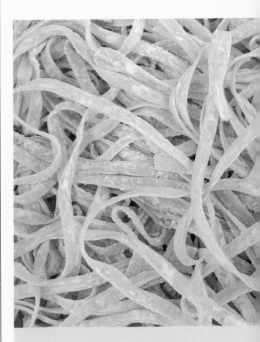

▲ Noodles are popular all over Asia. They are sometimes fried in oil as a snack.

Meals with grains

The third step in building a balanced diet based on grains is to try and introduce grains into every meal. Here are some tasty ways to do so.

Breakfast

Grains and breakfast go together naturally. Porridge, cornflakes or other cereals with low-fat milk are a great way to start the day. If your favourite brands use refined grains or have lots of sugar and salt, mix in a little wholegrain cereal such as shredded wheat, oats or some muesli.

For variety, try yogurt instead of milk. Adding fruit – strawberries, blueberries, peaches, raisins, sliced banana – to your cereal will also increase the nutritional value.

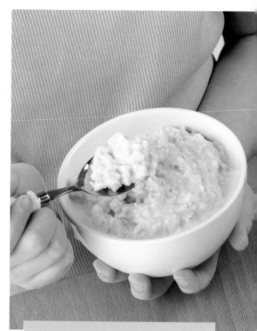

▲ A bowl of cereal such as porridge is a good way to start your day with eating whole grains.

Nutrition facts

Changing grains for better nutrients

instead of	try
white rice	wild rice, millet, quinoa, or couscous (coarsely ground millet or wheat)
white flour	wholemeal flour, wheat germ, or oats
potato crisps	rice cakes or popcorn (see popped amaranth recipe on page 22)
white pastas	wholegrain pastas (see page 11)
white breads	wholemeal or multigrain breads (see page 21)
chips	polenta wedges (see recipe on page 18)

Lunch ideas

For lunch, choose wholemeal or multigrain breads and pittas. You can dip the breads into olive oil flavoured with herbs as an alternative to butter. Grains can also be made into salads, as discussed on page 15. Mix bulgur with tomatoes, mint, spring onions and olive oil.

Rice cakes or crackers, corn crisps and water biscuits are satisfyingly crunchy and offer you better nutrition than sugary snacks. Adding cheese, cream cheese or hummus can boost nutrition and flavour.

What is for dinner?

For dinner, eat brown rice, millet, bulgur or couscous instead of white rice. Add whole grains, such as barley, amaranth or quinoa, to soups. Use wholegrain pastas, or try polenta instead. Because grains have plenty of bulk, you might eat less meat without even noticing it. You can even mix grains into your mince. It will have the same flavour but it will be better for you.

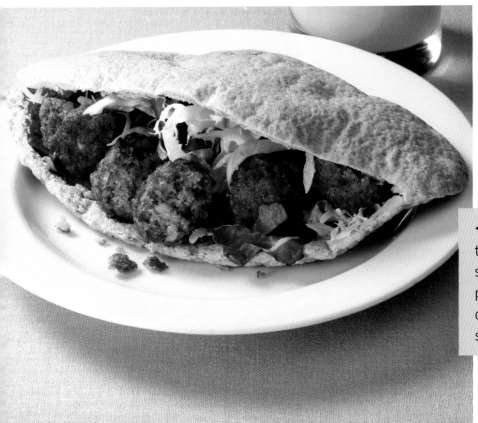

Recipe

Spiced pitta crisps

Makes 64 crisps.
Ingredients
4 wholemeal pitta breads
olive oil (approx. 30ml)
any herbs and spices (try curry
    powder; oregano and thyme;
    or black pepper)

Preparation
Preheat the oven to 180°C (Gas
    mark 4). Lightly oil a baking
    tray.
Using scissors, cut round the
    outside of each pitta to separate
    its layers. With a pastry brush,
    cover each pitta lightly with oil.
    Stack the pittas then cut down
    through the stack as if you were
    slicing a pie into eight pieces.
Spread the pitta triangles on a
    baking tray in a single layer.
    Sprinkle the triangles with your
    choice of spices.
Bake for 5 to 10 minutes or until
    golden. Allow the crisps to cool
    before eating or storing them.

◀ Pitta bread is ideal for filling, too. Split each pitta down one side to make a pocket. Fill the pocket with falafel, meat, salad, dip or spread – or a mixture of some of these.

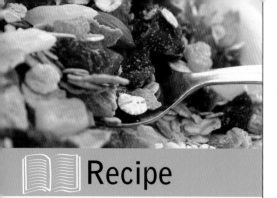

Polenta pizza faces

Makes 8 servings.
Ingredients
160g polenta meal
1l water
250g grated cheddar cheese
215ml pizza sauce
assorted fresh vegetables: try
   sliced black olives, sliced
   mushrooms, sliced red pepper,
   broccoli florets, chopped onions
sunflower oil (approx. 10ml)

Preparation
Preheat the oven to 190°C (Gas
   mark 5). Lightly oil two baking
   sheets with the sunflower oil.
Bring the water to the boil, then
   turn down the heat. Stir
   constantly while slowly adding
   the polenta meal in a thin,
   steady stream. Continue stirring
   to avoid lumps until the mixture
   is thick (2 to 5 minutes). Stir in
   125g of the grated cheese.
Make four polenta circles on each
   sheet, spreading them into flat
   pancake shapes about 15cm
   across.
Spread a layer of pizza sauce over
   each polenta circle. Top with the
   remaining cheese. Use the
   vegetables to create faces. Bake
   for 15 to 20 minutes, or until
   bubbly.

Vegetarian meals

So far, you have taken three steps towards building a balanced diet. First, you adjusted the portions of foods from different groups. Second, you started eating some whole grains. Both of these improved the nutrients you get. Third, you began exploring the variety of grains, to get a good mix of flavours and textures.

A fourth step – cutting out meat

If you eat meat regularly, try avoiding it for at least one dinner a week. Just switching from red meat to fish or poultry several times a week will improve your diet by reducing the amount of animal fat you eat. A diet with no meat at all can be even more healthy.

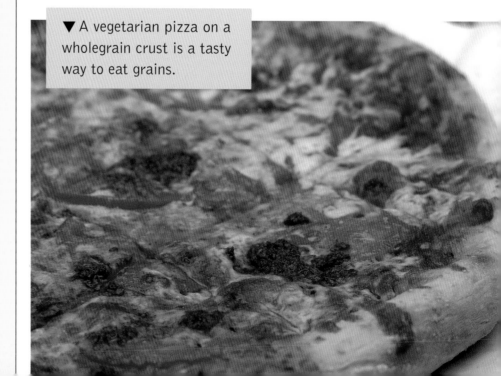

▼ A vegetarian pizza on a wholegrain crust is a tasty way to eat grains.

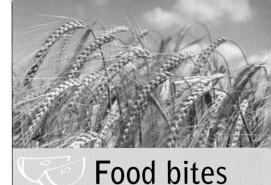

The meat-free diet

People who eat no meat – red or white – are known as vegetarians. Some vegetarians will eat fish as they do not think of it as 'meat'. People who eat no animal foods at all – meat, fish, eggs, cheese or milk – are known as vegans. Dietary variety is especially important for vegetarians and even more so for vegans.

Getting a good variety

One advantage of animal-based foods is that they give you all the kinds of protein you need in one convenient package. If you do not eat meat, you have to depend on a variety of foods to give you all your proteins.

Various combinations of grains, nuts and pulses – dried beans, peas and lentils – can supply everything you need. For example, grains are low in the amino acid lysine. But beans are rich in lysine, so if you include both in your diet, you get a more complete protein.

Nutrition facts

Veggie options

Grains and other sources of nutrients found in meat:

calcium: bread and breakfast cereals, soya milk, orange juice, dairy products, watercress, broccoli, sardines

iron: bread and breakfast cereals, nuts, tomato juice, rice, tofu, lentils, beans, apricots, eggs

zinc: whole grains, eggs, dairy products, nuts, tofu, leafy and root vegetables

vitamin B1: breakfast cereals, milk, eggs, fruit and vegetables

vitamin E: breakfast cereals, bread, vegetable oils, eggs

Food bites

Grains for snacks

Wheat, oats, barley and rye are used to make all kinds of crackers, breadsticks, crispbreads, flatbreads, pretzels and water biscuits. These are great for dipping into vegetable dips and spreads. Pretzels are thin, crisp breadsticks often made in the shape of a knot.

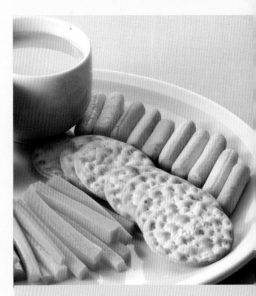

▲ Water biscuits and breadsticks are great for dips.

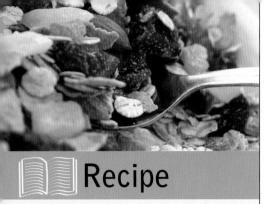

Chicken-noodle salad

Makes 6 servings.

Ingredients

250g-packet buckwheat noodles
45ml rice vinegar
35ml soy sauce
45ml sunflower oil
25ml sesame oil
1 walnut-size piece fresh ginger,
   grated
2 skinless, boneless chicken
   breasts, cooked and shredded
   (approx. 250g)
1 stalk celery, chopped
$1/2$ large sweet, red pepper,
   chopped
250g seedless green grapes
75g slivered almonds
100g mung bean sprouts

Preparation

Cook the noodles according to the
   instructions on the packet.
Meanwhile, mix the vinegar, soy
   sauce, oils and ginger in the
   bottom of a big bowl.
When the noodles are cooked,
   rinse them in cold water, drain
   and add to the bowl.
Toss the noodles well. Add the
   chicken, vegetables, grapes, nuts
   and sprouts. Toss and serve.

Cooking and serving

G rains are easy to cook. They are also lightweight and easy to carry and store. This makes them ideal foods the world over. People realised this in ancient times, too. Once humans discovered that you could plant grains, grow them in fields and cook them easily, it was possible to create farms and communities.

Cooking grains

To cook most grains, simply put them in a saucepan, add boiling water, cover the pan, lower the heat and simmer. Cooking times vary from 10 to 60 minutes depending

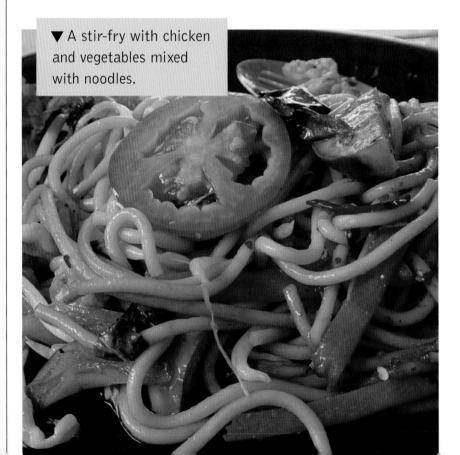

▼ A stir-fry with chicken and vegetables mixed with noodles.

on the grain. While white rice cooks in about 15 minutes, buckwheat, bulgur, polenta, couscous, rolled oats and rye are ready in 10 minutes. For a richer flavour, start by heating a little oil in the saucepan. Add the dry grain and stir for a minute or two before adding boiling water.

Grains such as bulgur and couscous should be soaked in hot water rather than cooked over heat. Put the grains in a heat-proof bowl, add boiling water, cover and let it stand for 10 minutes.

Grains can also be cooked in a steamer or pressure cooker. Steaming is a good way to keep in the nutrients.

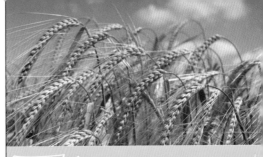

Food bites

Extra flavour

Grains need not be eaten plain.
- Cook them in chicken or vegetable stock.
- Add a little soy sauce, miso or Marmite.
- Grate some cheese on top.
- Add herbs such as dill or basil.
- Add sautéed vegetables or chopped onions and a little olive oil.
- Add curry powder, nuts and raisins.

You can even mix grains, for example rice and oats or bulgur. Cook the grains separately if the cooking times differ. Mix them when they are done, and serve hot or cold.

Nutrition facts

Baking bread

Most breads are baked in an oven. This can be a gas or electric oven at home or in a factory, or in an outdoor clay oven heated with hot charcoal. Flatbreads may be grilled, heated on a hot plate or baked in an oven. Bread fresh from the oven and still warm is particularly tasty. Cooled bread can be eaten as it is or toasted, grilled or fried. There are recipes for breads on some of the websites listed on page 31.

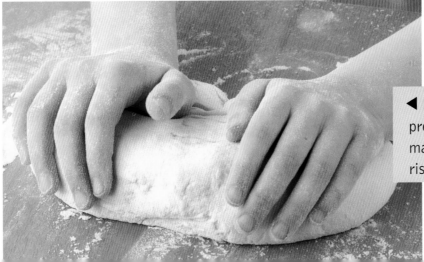

◀ Bread dough is kneaded, or pressed and stretched, to make it smooth and to help it rise when baked.

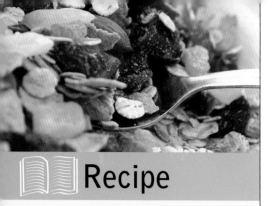

Chocolate happiness

Makes about 24 bars.
Ingredients
70g amaranth
5g unsweetened cocoa powder
150ml honey
15g unsalted butter
40ml rapeseed oil

Preparation
Lightly oil a 15 x 26cm baking
   tray.
Have an adult pop the amaranth
   just like popcorn, a tablespoon
   at a time. Add it to a very hot,
   heavy frying pan. Cover and
   shake the pan until the grains
   pop – about 10 seconds. Transfer
   the grains to a bowl. Repeat
   until all the grains are done.
Add the cocoa powder and mix.
Combine the remaining ingredients
   in a heavy-bottomed pan and
   bring to the boil. Reduce the
   heat to medium and cook,
   stirring constantly, until the
   mixture thickens (8 to 10
   minutes). Pour the mixture over
   the amaranth.
Mix well. Press the mixture into
   the prepared baking tray,
   smoothing the top with a
   spatula.
Cut into bars and allow to cool.
   The bars may be stored in an
   air-tight container.

Digestion

Your body cannot use the nutrients in grains and other foods until it separates them and carries them to cells. The first part of this process is digestion. This begins with chewing. With your teeth, you cut up and mash food into pieces small enough to swallow. Chewing also mixes the food with chemicals, called enzymes, in your saliva. These start dissolving the food. When you swallow, the food is pushed down a tube, the oesophagus, towards your stomach.

The digestive tube

In your stomach, strong chemicals and more enzymes go to work on the food. The partly digested food then travels to the intestines. There, proteins are broken into tinier pieces called amino acids, carbohydrates into glucose, and fats into smaller chemical units known as glycerol and fatty acids.

All these nutrients, along with vitamins and minerals, pass out of the digestive tube into the lymph and blood systems for processing, mainly in the liver.

Nutrition facts

All kinds of sugar
During digestion, carbohydrates in grains and other foods are broken down into a simple sugar, glucose. Other common sugars that appear in grain products include corn sweetener, corn syrup, dextrose, maltose, mannitol and sorbitol.

The digestive system

A 10-m-long tube

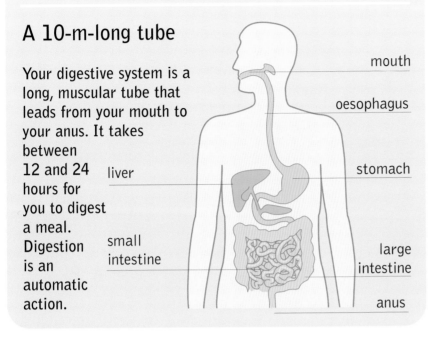

Your digestive system is a long, muscular tube that leads from your mouth to your anus. It takes between 12 and 24 hours for you to digest a meal. Digestion is an automatic action.

mouth

oesophagus

liver

stomach

small intestine

large intestine

anus

Whatever is left over is now pushed out of the body, helped along by the fibre you have eaten. You cannot control digestion, but when your stomach is empty you feel hungry. When you have eaten enough, you start to feel full. This can be uncomfortable when you have eaten too much. Only eat as much as you need.

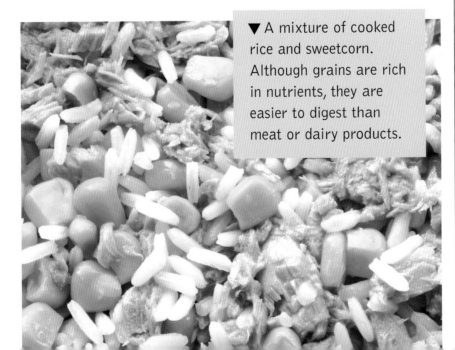

▼ A mixture of cooked rice and sweetcorn. Although grains are rich in nutrients, they are easier to digest than meat or dairy products.

Food bites

Food allergies

Sometimes, a person's body reacts as if a particular food were attacking it, like a virus or a poison. Eating a food you are allergic to may make you itchy, feel sick or have trouble breathing.

Some people's digestive systems cannot handle gluten, a protein found in wheat. This is known as coeliac disease. Sufferers must avoid wheat, rye, oats and barley, but can eat rice, maize, millet, buckwheat and some of the less familiar grains. Some manufacturers of bread, cakes and biscuits also make special gluten-free foods for people with coeliac disease.

A day's worth of energy

kcal	meals
	breakfast
156	2 boiled eggs
69	1 orange
130	2 pieces wholewheat toast
102	1 glass semi-skimmed milk
	lunch
73	bowl of mushroom and barley soup
80	green, leafy salad with oil and vinegar
154	1 glass grape juice
112	1 oatmeal biscuit
	snack
234	2 rice cakes with 2 slices mozzarella cheese
110	1 apple
	dinner
233	1 small piece grilled salmon
166	1 cup wild rice
54	1 cup steamed carrots
65	1 slice multigrain bread
258	1 small scoop ice-cream and 1 spoon fudge sauce
1,996	**GRAND TOTAL**

Energy balance

If you eat a balanced diet and exercise regularly, you will look and feel good. You will get as much energy from foods and drinks as you need. Grain foods, having lots of carbohydrates, provide most of your energy. Pasta is a particular favourite of athletes as it releases energy over a long period of time.

Exactly how much energy you need depends on your age, gender and how active you are. If you eat more kilocalories than your body can use, the extra energy is stored as fat. Having too much body fat, or being overweight, can create health problems.

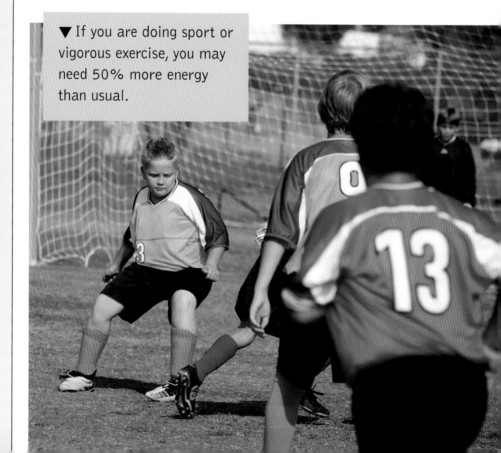

▼ If you are doing sport or vigorous exercise, you may need 50% more energy than usual.

Body Mass Index

Your Body Mass Index (BMI) is a number that shows how your weight compares to your height. Doctors and dieticians use the BMI as a guide to your health. Your BMI percentile (a word from 'per cent') tells you how you compare to everyone else of your age and sex. If your BMI percentile is between 5% and 85%, you are in the normal range. You are probably getting a good balance of food and exercise. You can work out your BMI percentile using a calculator on some of the websites listed on page 31. Ordinary height and weight charts, like those below, are also good guides to normal growth and development.

Weight control

The simplest way to control your weight is to avoid saturated fats. Grains are low in kilocalories but what you eat with them may not be. Cut down on the amount of butter you eat on bread and the cheese on your pasta. Choosing whole grains over refined grains will help too. These are better ways than 'going on a diet'.

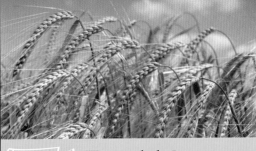

Food bites

Daily energy needs

Children aged 7-10:
about 2,000 kcal
Girls aged 11-14:
about 2,200 kcal
Boys aged 11-14:
about 2,500 kcal
If you want to count calories in foods, you can look them up on food labels, or on the Internet. But you should not need to do this if your diet is balanced.
1 kcal = 4.2 kJ

Average weight

Choose the correct chart. For your age, see where you are on the graph. If your weight is near to the red line marking the average weight, that is fine. If not, you may need to balance your diet more carefully.

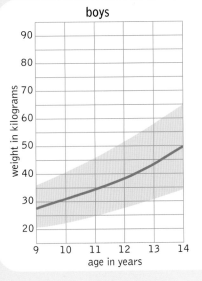

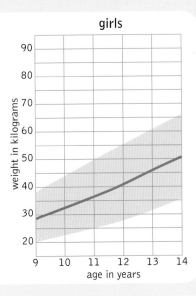

Storing grains

Uncooked grains will keep well for a few months in glass or plastic jars kept in a cool, dry place. Those grains that are high in oils, such as millet, will eventually go stale, but you can easily tell if that has happened by smelling them.

Shopping and storing

There is one more important step to building a balanced diet: sensible food shopping. With grain products, as with other foods, buy fresh and natural produce when you can. The more ready-made or prepared a product is, the more things have been added to it so that it can be stored longer or cooked faster. These foods are convenient, but should not be a major part of your diet.

When you are buying breads, pastas, breakfast cereals or grains, always look for wholemeal products. They contain all the nutrients of the original grains.

▶ Most supermarkets and health food shops now sell a wide range of grains. Next time you go food shopping, look for some unusual grains to get your family to try.

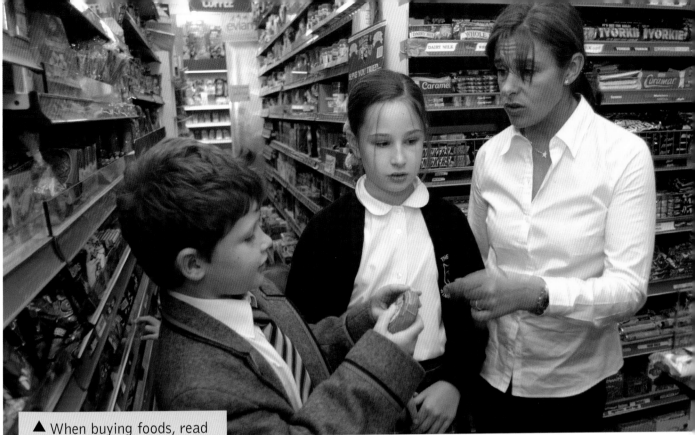

▲ When buying foods, read the labels carefully for ingredients and nutrient and calorie contents.

However, some refined-grain breakfast cereals and breads are 'fortified' or enriched. Vitamins and minerals have been added to them, often to restore some of the nutrients lost in refining. These grain foods lack bran (fibre) but still have nutritional value. Yet other products have added bran but are not wholegrain.

Look at the label

Most food packaging has labels not only listing the ingredients but also stating what percentage of your recommended daily amounts (RDA) for each nutrient a portion contains. You can use these figures to help balance your diet. Labels on grain foods often also show if the product is wholegrain, enriched, gluten-free and suitable for vegetarians and vegans.

Nutrition facts

Shelf life

Grain foods such as bread, pasta and cakes are often mass-produced using additives. These are chemicals added to improve the texture and shelf life of the foods. Grain foods that have 'gone off' quickly become covered in moulds. You should not eat foods past their 'use by' date. If you do, you could get a stomach upset.

Cooking safety

Here are some rules you should follow when cooking and making recipes.

- ask an adult for permission to cook and for help in handling anything sharp or hot
- wash your hands before you begin
- after handling raw meat, wash your hands, cooking tools and surfaces with hot, soapy water
- wash fruits and vegetables before using
- use pot holders or oven gloves when handling something hot
- keep saucepan handles turned towards the back of the stove
- open saucepan lids away from you to avoid burning your face with steam
- avoid loose, long sleeves, or roll them up
- keep your fingers and hair out of the way when using appliances
- never plug in appliances with wet hands

Projects

Here are some ideas for things you can do related to grains and diet. Discover the variety of grains that is available. Record what you are eating now and see how you can introduce more grains into a balanced diet.

Action 1

Supermarket detective

- How many different kinds of grains can you find in your local supermarket? How many different kinds of rice?
- Write down the price of the same weight of five wholegrain products. Compare the price of the same weight of five non-grain foods. Check the labels for fibre, kilocalories, fat, sugar and salt content. Create a graph of this information.
- Take a look at the pasta and cereals sections in the supermarket. How many different kinds of grains can you find listed as ingredients?
- Now look at the ready-made foods section. How many of these grains can you find listed as ingredients? Are there more or fewer than you imagined?
- How many of the foods contain genetically modified grains? This should be clearly marked on the labels.

Food tracking

Make a chart like the one shown below. Keep a list for five days of everything you eat. Then put a tick for each item into the appropriate box. (Some foods will need more than one tick.) Count the number of ticks in each category and write the totals in the right-hand column.

	Monday	Tuesday	Wednesday	Thursday	Friday	TOTAL
whole grains						
refined grains						
fruits						
vegetables						
nuts or seeds						
pulses						
red meat						
poultry						
seafood						
dairy foods						
junk foods						

- How many whole grains did you eat compared with refined grains?
- Which category of food did you eat the most?
- Create a new chart for another five days. Before you use the chart, think of ways to make your diet more balanced. Use some of the ideas in this book.
- Compare the two charts. Have any of the categories of food become more or less important in your diet?

Make a grains chart

Make a chart with a column for each of the grains mentioned in this book. Make rows for the size, colour and shape of the grains and which countries they come from.

Leave a space at the top of each column to glue a small sample of the grain.

See how many of the grains you have at home. See how many more you can find at your local supermarket or store. If you can, glue a sample of each grain on to your chart. What are the similarities and differences between the grains? Do more of them come from Asia and Africa than from the rest of the world? Why do you think this is?

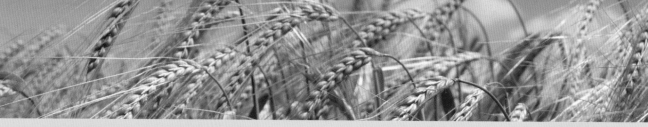

Glossary

CARBOHYDRATES
One of the three main nutrients in food. They are made of sugar molecules and mostly provide energy.

DIET
The food and drink that a person eats.

EDIBLE
What you can eat safely.

ENZYMES
Substances that help digestion and other chemical processes.

FATS
One of the three main nutrients in food. They are made of fatty acids and glycerol and mostly provide an energy store.

GLUTEN
A protein, mostly in wheat, that some people are allergic to.

GRAINS
The edible seeds of grass plants.

INGREDIENTS
Individual items of food that are required to make a particular dish.

KILOCALORIES
The units used to measure the energy in food and drink.

LYMPH SYSTEM
A circulation system that carries nutrients from digestion round the body.

MINERALS
Nutrients needed for health. They include iron, calcium, sodium and zinc.

NUTRIENTS
Materials the body needs but cannot make itself.

NUTRITIONAL VALUE
How rich or poor a food or drink is in nutrients.

OILS
Fats that are naturally liquid.

POULTRY
Birds kept for meat and eggs, in particular chickens, turkeys and ducks. Their meat is called 'white meat' to contrast with red meat.

PROTEINS
One of the three main nutrients in food. They are made of amino acids and mostly provide building materials for the body.

RED MEAT
Meat rich in blood, in particular beef, lamb, veal, pork and venison.

SIMMER
To cook in a liquid that is hot but not quite boiling.

STAPLE
A food that forms a large part of people's diet.

VITAMINS
Nutrients needed in small quantities for health, fitness and body processes.

WHOLEGRAIN
Grain including the outer bran.

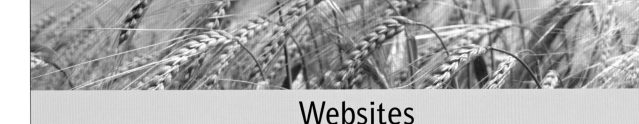

Websites

Here is a selection of websites that have information and activities about grains, diet, health and fitness.

http://www.breakfastcereal.org/
A wide variety of information about breakfast cereals.

http://www.mypyramid.gov/pyramid/
   grains.html
Facts, figures and information about grains and how they fit in the food pyramid and a balanced diet.

http://www.kelloggs.co.uk/health/
General science and diet information about grains. Includes fun activities.

http://www.baking911.com/bread/101
   _intro.htm
Gives detailed information, tips, techniques and simple recipes for baking all kinds of bread.

http://www.msgtruth.org/msgand2.htm
Information about gluten and a gluten-free diet.

http://dmoz.org/Home/Cooking/Grains/
Provides information about cooking grains, plus lots of recipes.

http://www.vegsoc.org/info/cereals.
   html
Information about cereals specifically for vegetarians.

http://www.eatwell.gov.uk/info/games/
Games and activities about food and diet from the government's Food Standards Agency.

http://www.healthchoice.org.uk/
   fortified/default.aspx
Gives information on fortified foods.

http://www.foodafactoflife.org.uk/
Educational material about food, diet and nutrients.

http://www.blubberbuster.com/height_
   weight.html
Allows you to calculate your body mass index.

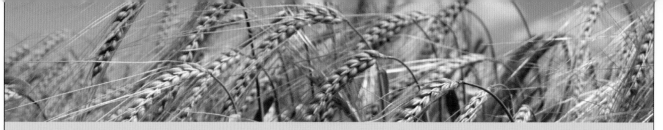

Index

amaranth 12, 13, 15, 17, 22

barley 4, 9, 12, 13, 15, 17, 19, 23
biscuits 4, 17, 19, 23
bran 5, 11
bread 4, 6, 7, 8, 10, 11, 13, 15, 16, 17, 19, 21, 23, 24, 25, 26, 27, 30
buckwheat 13, 23

cakes 10, 11, 24, 27
calories and kilocalories 5, 6, 9, 10, 11, 24, 25, 27, 28, 30
carbohydrates 4, 6, 8, 9, 22, 24, 30
cereals 4, 7, 9, 10, 12, 14, 16, 19, 26, 27, 28
corn 13, 17, 22
couscous 17, 21

dairy products 4, 7, 19, 23, 29
diet 4, 5, 6, 7, 11, 16, 18, 24, 25, 26, 28, 30
digestion and digestive system 4, 9, 22, 23, 30

eggs 7, 11, 15, 19, 24
energy 4, 5, 8, 9, 24, 30
exercise 4, 5, 6, 24

fats 4, 6, 5, 10, 11, 18, 22, 24, 25, 28, 30
fibre 4, 8, 9, 10, 28
flour 5, 10, 11, 12, 13, 15, 16
food allergies 23

genetically modified (GM) foods 12, 28
germ 5, 11, 16
gluten 23, 30

maize 12, 13, 15, 23
meat 4, 7, 11, 14, 15, 17, 18, 19, 23, 28, 29, 30
millet 12, 13, 15, 16, 17, 23, 26
minerals 4, 6, 8, 22, 27, 30
muesli 10, 16

noodles 4, 11, 14, 15, 20
nutrients 4, 6, 7, 9, 11, 13, 18, 22, 23, 27, 29, 30

oats 4, 9, 12, 13, 15, 16, 19, 21, 23
oils 12, 17, 18, 19, 20, 21, 22, 24, 29, 30

pasta 4, 7, 9, 10, 11, 16, 17, 24, 25, 27, 28
polenta 16, 17, 18
porridge 10, 16

proteins 4, 6, 7, 8, 10, 19, 22, 30

quinoa 12, 13, 14, 15, 16, 17

rice 4, 5, 7, 17, 19, 20, 23, 24
rye 12, 13, 15, 19, 21, 23

salt 5, 8, 15, 16, 28
seeds 4, 5, 29, 30
sorghum 12, 13
steps to a balanced diet 7, 11, 16, 18, 26
sugars and starches 4, 5, 8, 9, 11, 16, 22, 28, 30
sweetcorn 8, 13, 21, 23

triticale 12, 13

vegetables 6, 7, 11, 14, 19, 20, 21, 28, 29
vegetarian and vegan 18–19, 27
vitamins 4, 6, 8, 22, 27, 30

water 6, 8, 9, 10, 11, 14, 15, 17, 20, 29
wheat 4, 7, 10, 11, 12, 13, 15, 16, 19, 21, 23, 30
wholegrain and wholemeal 5, 7, 10, 11, 16, 17, 18, 19, 25, 26, 27, 30

PRESTON COLLEGE
WILLIAM TUSON LIBRARY